What a Teenager & His Mom Want You to Know about Preventing & Recovering from Concussions

HEADSTRONG

BY LUKE AND MYRA HEAVNER

Copyright © 2018 by Myra and Luke Heavner

All rights reserved. This book may not be reproduced or stored in whole or in part by any means without the written permission of the author except for brief quotations for the purpose of review.

ISBN: 978-1-943258-86-4

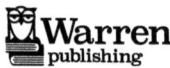

Published by Warren Publishing
Charlotte, NC
www.warrenpublishing.net
Printed in the United States

*In memory of all who suffered
from concussions in silence,
and in honor of those who
are still recovering.*

*A special thanks from Myra to Dr. Joey Miles,
Dr. Jason Glass, Travis Glass, Sight Works,
and David R. Wiercisiewski, MD,
Deanna Dunn and Angel Watson.*

FOREWORD

For many years now, I have worked with patients experiencing vision disturbances and visual processing delays after an injury. Patients present with very similar subjective symptoms regardless of age and incident particulars. However, the same type of traumatic event may have a drastically different visual effect on different individuals. In some concussion patients, the visual system is not affected in any way. Often patients are desperately seeking some explanation for what they are experiencing. Their symptoms which can be frustrating to articulate, especially when all functional testing shows normal results. Patients don't feel "normal" in any way, which can compound their emotional distress.

The brain is a miraculous organ that we don't fully understand due to it's amazing complexity. I am so thankful that Luke and Myra have been willing to share their very personal experiences. For years, I have asked patients to share their experiences in an effort to help others walking through similar life challenges. By the time I encounter many patients, they feel desperate, alone, and anxious because they are not sure what to do next. Luke's description provides a glimpse into his real and raw emotions as he walked through this hardship. His situation is far more common than one would expect.

I have enjoyed caring for Luke over many years as his primary eye care provider. When he presented to my office post-concussion, it was obvious that he was suffering from the visual side effects associated with a traumatic brain injury. He expressed many symptoms that we repeatedly hear from our concussion patients.

As a parent myself, I can understand the helplessness felt when you are not sure how to move forward with your child. It is confusing when there is no hard physical explanation for such a drastic change in your child's behavior. Myra has done a beautiful job sharing her feelings as a mom and providing encouragement to others. Their story will most definitely help others navigate the tumultuous waters of a concussion and, at minimum, provide reassurance that many others have experienced something similar. Thank you, Luke and Myra, for sharing your story!

Amanda Barker Assell, O.D.

PART I
LUKE HEAVNER

A TEEN'S CONCUSSION STORY

Hi, my name is Luke, and I live with my parents in a small city in North Carolina called Lincolnton.

I'm fourteen, and like many kids my age, I like to play video games, hang out with my friends, hunt, fish, and play sports.

But there was a time I couldn't do what I wanted, and that's why my mom and I decided to write this book. You see, we want to share the story of what happened to me two and a half years ago when I was eleven and suffered a concussion—*two* concussions, actually—in less than two weeks.

We're sharing this story because we didn't know anything then about concussions. We wish we had. We wish we'd known sooner about things like concussion symptoms, the triggers for symptoms, the types of treatments, and the recovery outcomes.

I especially wish I had known how serious a concussion can be, and about what can happen when you don't pay attention to your body's distress signals. What I wish *most* of all, though, is for my story to help *you* identify the possibility

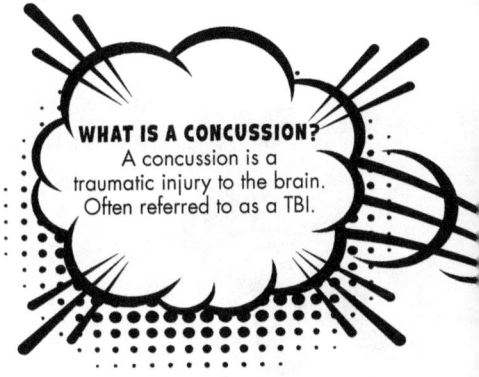

WHAT IS A CONCUSSION?
A concussion is a traumatic injury to the brain. Often referred to as a TBI.

of a concussion and how to avoid additional brain trauma while you're healing. And if you're currently recovering from a concussion, I hope my story will validate your feelings and experiences, because you are not alone, or going crazy.

But my story isn't meant to scare you. After all I'm here, writing this book with my mom. Instead, my story is meant to help you find the words and the strength to speak up for yourself if you suspect you have a concussion, or if you're ever diagnosed with one.

In other words, this is the book my parents and I wish we'd come across two years ago *before* my concussion injuries, and during the earliest phase of my recovery.

So, here's my story:

Two and a half years ago when I was eleven, I was at football practice in full pads when my teammate pulled my face mask. My feet fell out from underneath me and I felt a sharp twist in my neck as my head slammed into the ground. Right away, my head started hurting. When I got back on my feet, I could tell something wasn't right.

I felt different, but I didn't know then how to explain what I was feeling. That night after practice, I told my mom about the hit and that my head was hurting. Neither of us thought then about a concussion. We both thought I'd

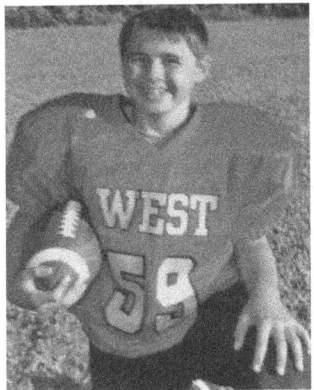
Luke, 11, in his football uniform before the concussion

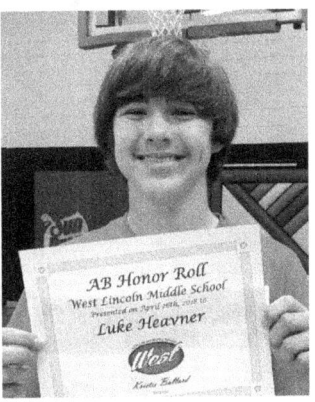
Luke, 14, after achieving the A/B Honor Roll in Middle School

feel better in the morning, but I didn't. I lay around, and was sleepy, and my headache got worse. I had a sore neck and jaw pain.

The next day was the third of a four-day event at my school for rising sixth graders—Jump Start. Even though my head was still hurting, I went anyway.

Everyone had to take a test that day, but getting through the test was much harder for me than usual. I couldn't concentrate and couldn't shake off the headache. All day, I felt as if I were moving in slow motion. All I wanted to do was sleep. On day four of Jump Start, I couldn't go. My head was hurting and I felt funny. That's the only way I could describe it at the time—*funny*. So I went back to bed and slept all day. I remember being really thirsty and very sleepy.

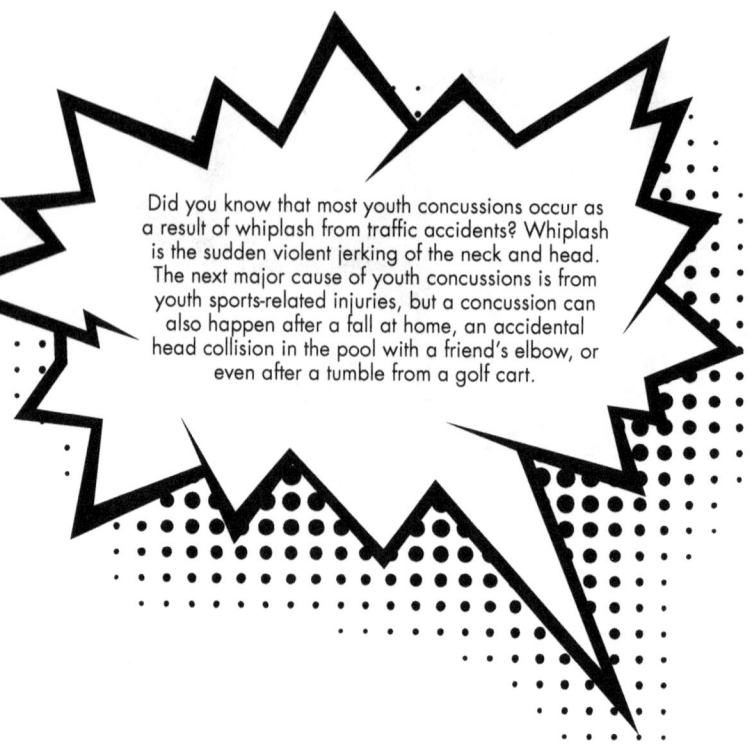

Did you know that most youth concussions occur as a result of whiplash from traffic accidents? Whiplash is the sudden violent jerking of the neck and head. The next major cause of youth concussions is from youth sports-related injuries, but a concussion can also happen after a fall at home, an accidental head collision in the pool with a friend's elbow, or even after a tumble from a golf cart.

On the morning of the third day after the hard hit during football practice, I told my parents that I needed to see a doctor. My dad drove me to our family doctor, and he was the first to tell us that I had a concussion. He said there was nothing I could do but rest until I was headache-free for twenty-four hours.

I didn't know what a concussion was back then. I had no idea that when you take a hard jolting tackle that suddenly changes the direction of your head and neck, or a direct blow to your head with the ground or with another helmet, these blows can actually cause your brain to slam against the inside of your skull. A concussion actually puts a bruise on your brain. The medical experts describe it like this: The inside of your skull is actually rough, not smooth like you might think. And since your brain isn't completely protected by a coating called myelin until you're about fourteen, every jolt you take can cause your brain to bang or rub against the rough inside part of your skull, causing tears to your brain tissue. These tears, depending on the severity and the location of them on the brain, can affect all sorts of things like your balance or your ability to think clearly, make you nervous, or sometimes even scared because you don't know what's going on inside your body. You suddenly just feel different.

Also, the sudden, violent jolt your brain takes inside your skull can set up a chemical chain reaction that makes it difficult for your brain to send the proper signals to the rest of your body. This difficulty can affect hand-eye coordination, balance, and ability to think clearly.

As I said, I didn't know any of this back then. Besides, everyone who heard about my concussion that day and afterward said the same thing: *You'll be fine in a day or two.* The doctor said to rest until I was headache-free for twenty-four hours straight, which at the time, sounded simple enough. But, who knew a headache could last for a year? For an eleven-year-old boy, following orders to rest isn't that easy when the rest restrictions include *no* TV, *no* phone, and *no* video games.

The first day or so of *rest* was fairly easy because all I wanted to do was sleep anyway. But when I was awake, the headaches returned, and I still felt as if I were moving in slow motion. When my mom called the doctor to explain that my headaches were getting worse, the doctor said there was nothing I could do but ride it out and *rest*. I couldn't get comfortable. I was crying because it was the worst headache I'd ever had, and it just wouldn't go away. Doctors will tell you that your brain tries to heal itself from the trauma and the tears, and the best way to help your brain

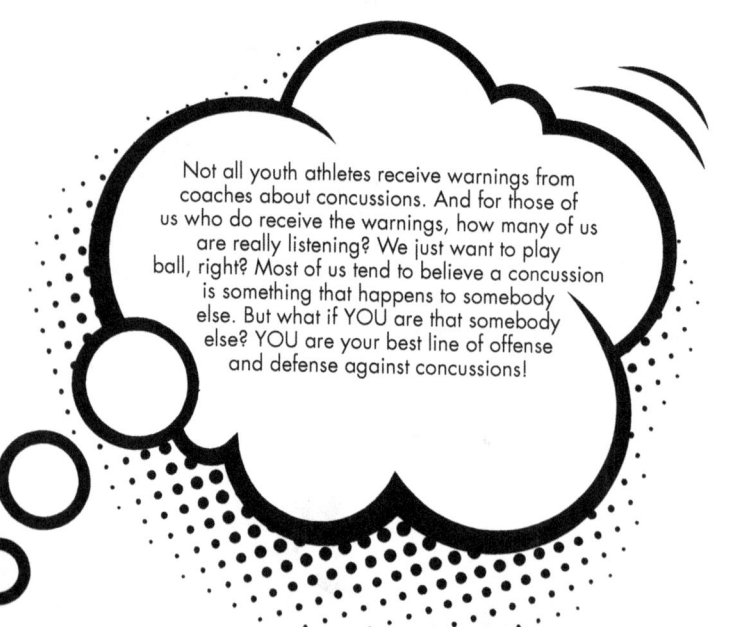

Not all youth athletes receive warnings from coaches about concussions. And for those of us who do receive the warnings, how many of us are really listening? We just want to play ball, right? Most of us tend to believe a concussion is something that happens to somebody else. But what if YOU are that somebody else? YOU are your best line of offense and defense against concussions!

heal itself is to let it rest during the healing process.

Sure, watching TV doesn't sound like it would be hard on your brain, but it is. And so is texting or concentrating on homework or tests. According to doctors, sometimes after a concussion, your brain has to rewire certain connections because of tissue tears or because of swollen and inflamed areas that have taken the heaviest blows against your skull.

> **CONCUSSION TIP #1**
> Don't try to resume any activities until you're headache-free for twenty-four hours!

Nine days later on August 21, the Friday before I was to start middle school, I was tired of lying around and doing nothing, so I told my mom I was feeling great—*even headache-free*—because school was starting Monday and I wanted to go fishing with friends that day. Of course, I still didn't feel right, but I kept quiet and managed to have fun that day.

The next day, I rode with a friend to weigh-in at football practice. I hadn't played since the hit, and I knew I couldn't play as long as the doctor felt I was supposed to be resting, but I wanted out of the house.

After the football weigh-in, my friend invited me to a birthday party, which sounded fun because I'd get to

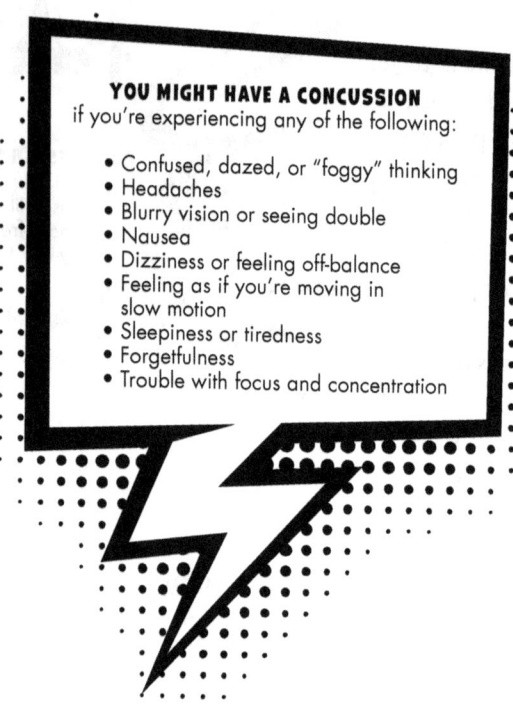

see all my friends I hadn't seen over the summer. The party also sounded like a great way to see everyone before the start of school on Monday. My parents let me go. After all, they thought I'd been headache-free for twenty-four hours.

At the party, we ran around and jumped on a trampoline. While wrestling with my friends, I got kicked in the head. Then, while jumping on the trampoline, I fell and hit my head *again*.

I didn't know then what additional blows to the head would do, *could do,* to a concussion that wasn't fully healed. Now I know those additional blows could have killed me, or put me at risk for permanent brain damage. At this point, I would live the next eighteen months in a dark, deep hole—all alone.

My life changed.

Instantly my brain felt like it was on fire. I was dizzy, and my eyes were seeing funny. By the time my mom picked me up, I was crying. I told my mom I had a fever and that my brain felt as if it were on fire. I didn't have a fever, but I did have a massive, burning headache. Once home, I went straight to bed. I didn't tell my parents I'd hit my head again, or that I'd been running around and jumping on the trampoline at the party. But everyone at the party knew I'd gotten hurt.

That Sunday at home, I was lying down but everything around me seemed like it was moving. My head was hurting worse than ever. I felt different, but I couldn't explain how. All I could do, and did, was sleep.

The next day was the first day of middle school—new school, teachers, and friends. I got ready for school, but I still felt weird. Still, I thought I could go, and that everything would be fine once I got there.

My mom drove me to school, but by the time we got there, my heart felt as if it were beating inside my head. My chest was pounding too, and my heart felt like it might explode. I started crying. "I can't get out of the car," I said to my mom, who looked at me with disbelief.

"It's your first day at school," she said. "Go on … get out."

"Mom, I can't. I feel like I'm having a heart attack," I cried.

She drove us straight to the emergency room. What I know now is that I was experiencing a panic attack. Panic attacks make you feel like you are having a heart attack and dying. My chest hurt. I had trouble breathing. I was sweating but cold, and I couldn't control my crying. I didn't understand why all of this was happening.

After an examination and tests, the ER doctor said I had a concussion. He said to rest, see a concussion specialist, and stay out of school until I was headache-free for twenty-four hours. He also gave us a six-stage plan called *Return to Learn* (see pages 32 and 33). The plan included a gradual move from one stage to the next.

A few days later, I saw a concussion specialist who told me to take the rest of the week off from school. He was a boxer and seemed to understand about blows to the head, and everything seemed like it would be okay. I was to return in six days.

I seemed fine over the Labor Day weekend. I took it easy and had a picnic on a boat with my family and friends. I still had the headache and a pressure inside my head as if it was full, or filling up with something. I also had the feeling of being off balance, but I was at home with no stress and didn't really have much to think about.

I thought everything was fine until Tuesday morning when it was time to return to school. I didn't want to go, and was crying because I felt so bad. But my parents insisted I had to go to school.

I was so confused about how bad I felt that I began to act out of character, even hiding under my bed to avoid going to school. When that didn't work, I hid under the car. And when that didn't work, either, I refused to get in the car. I had never acted like this before and I was scared. I'm sure my parents were too. Something inside my head didn't feel right and I didn't know how to describe the feeling to them.

My parents forced me to go to school, but I left early that day to follow up with the concussion specialist. He gave me tests on my memory. I couldn't pass any of his tests, like remembering three numbers.

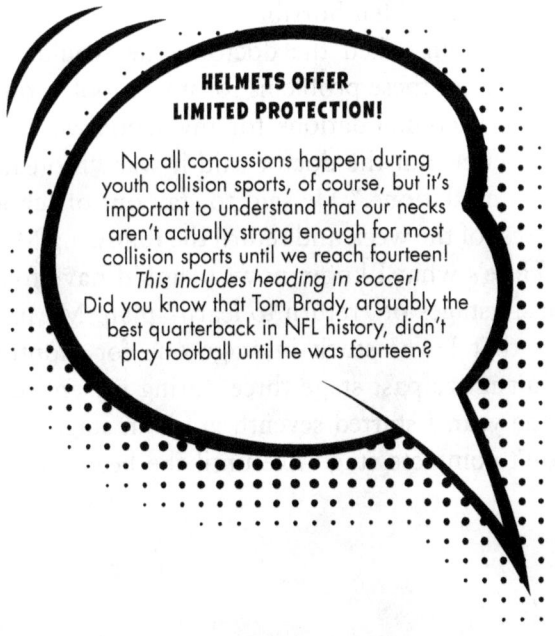

HELMETS OFFER LIMITED PROTECTION!

Not all concussions happen during youth collision sports, of course, but it's important to understand that our necks aren't actually strong enough for most collision sports until we reach fourteen! *This includes heading in soccer!* Did you know that Tom Brady, arguably the best quarterback in NFL history, didn't play football until he was fourteen?

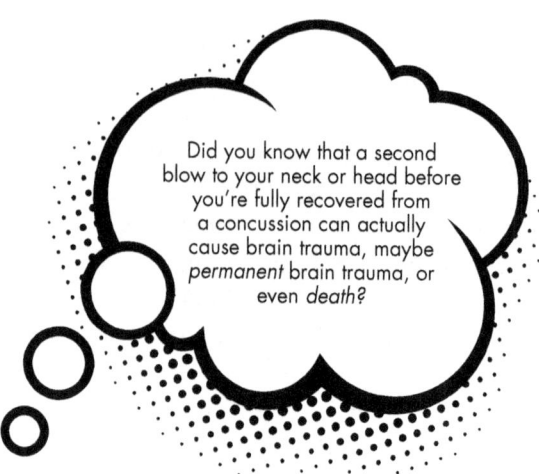

I couldn't even follow the movement of his fingers. The doctor wrote a prescription for attention deficit medication to see if this would help with my lack of concentration and focus. I was seeing double, however, and I felt horrible.

My mom asked the doctor if he would write a letter about these problems for my school, requesting special accommodations for my schoolwork until I was better. But the doctor said it was "too early for accommodations." He said to stay out of school for the rest of the week and return the following Monday.

Here's what I know now: I should have followed the six stages of "return to learn" plan. My problem was that I was stuck in stage one for months and didn't move past stage three during my entire sixth-grade year. I started seventh grade in stage four and didn't complete stage five until the beginning of my eighth-grade year. Schools now have a "return-to-learn" policy like the one the emergency room gave us. When I was first recovering from my concussion, however, there was only a "return-to-play" policy in effect.

Monday came, and my headache seemed to get worse. My heart started to race again too, and I was scared—very scared. I wanted to die rather than return to school. The work was hard. It would take me twenty minutes to do ten easy math problems. I couldn't take notes or keep up with the work. I couldn't even write.

My parents and teachers thought I simply didn't want to go to school. But I was experiencing a pain I didn't know how to describe. All I could say was, "I don't know what's wrong with me." My parents thought they were helping by making me go to school. The school's guidance counselors also said things like, "Luke looks fine;" and, "If Luke can get a week under his belt and push through, the anxieties will go away;" and, "It's normal when you start middle school to have anxieties."

I didn't even know what anxieties were. What I did know was that the school was *so* loud. The lights were *so* bright. I couldn't keep up with what the teachers were saying. I felt as if I were moving in slow motion. The lunch room was unbearable. The noise was driving me crazy.

When I called my parents to ask them to pick me up, they said "no."

I asked my friends to call my parents for me.

I asked my teachers to let me go home.

Nobody would get me out of there, and I felt trapped. No one knew what I was feeling and I didn't know how to tell them. All I could do was cry.

Somehow, I made it through each day, but I would cry from the time I got home until it was time to go to school again. Then I'd follow the same routine for a couple more days. I was begging and crying not to go to school. All I could say was, "I'm scared." After I got to school, I would text my parents thirty to forty times an hour, begging them to pick me up. The ADD medication seemed to be making me more anxious, too, and I stopped taking it soon after.

One day as I got ready for school, I told my mom, "My head hurts so bad, I want to kill myself!" We ended up back in the emergency room. The experience was horrible because everyone wanted to help, but I couldn't explain the problem. The doctors gave me something to sleep and I felt so good because I had not been sleeping. When the doctors woke me up and wanted me to talk to a psychiatrist via Skype, I went crazy, kicking and screaming, because they'd interrupted my first real rest in a long time.

In the room with me was a security guard. My mom was told to leave, and when she was gone, the doctors explained that if it was true about me wanting to kill myself, they would have to take me from my parents for several weeks. I wouldn't be able to see them.

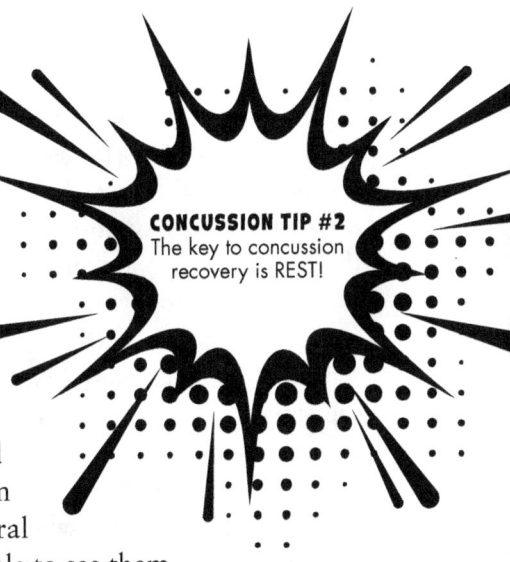

CONCUSSION TIP #2
The key to concussion recovery is REST!

I know now threatening to kill oneself is a very serious comment and doctors have to take this seriously to protect you from harm. So, I said I was lying. They called my mom back to the room. I was so happy when she said, "We can work on telling a lie, but we can't fix death." I love my parents and didn't want to be separated from them. I was just tired of my head hurting and of feeling weird all the time. The doctors may have admitted me to the hospital kicking and screaming, but I didn't have to stay overnight. The ER doctors gave me a note to stay out of school and encouraged me to meet with our family doctor. We came up with a plan that was supposed to help me gradually return to school. I was still expected to go, but according to the doctors' note, I was to be allowed to lay my head down, or do anything necessary to make myself comfortable.

But laying your head down at school doesn't work. For starters, no one understands or appreciates what it's like to be different. At school, you're supposed to do your work, pay attention, and act like the rest of the kids. I was no longer acting like I used to.

I continued to try at school, but I couldn't keep my end of the bargain with the doctor about our half-day school attendance plan. I couldn't stand to be there—the noise, the lights, the people, the work, and the computers all made me dizzy. I also had problems with my eyes—like double vision. Words on paper appeared to move around. The whole world, it seemed, was moving so fast, yet I was moving *sooooooooooooooo sloooooooooooooowly*. When I wasn't at school facing the mental stress of classwork, surrounded by people, and under bright lights, I felt better. Looking back

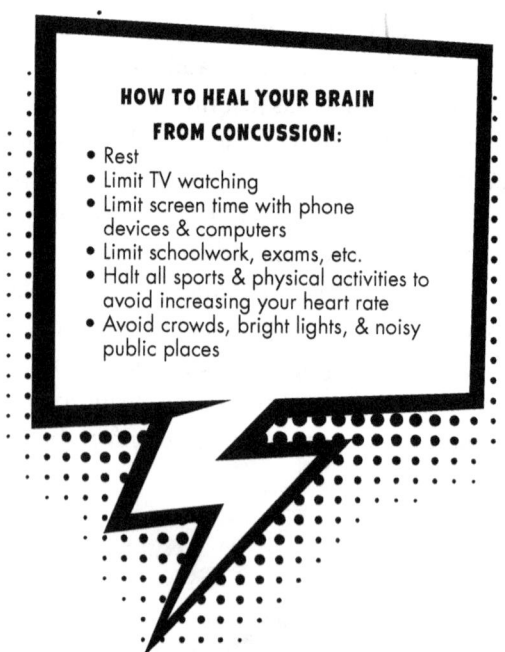

HOW TO HEAL YOUR BRAIN FROM CONCUSSION:
- Rest
- Limit TV watching
- Limit screen time with phone devices & computers
- Limit schoolwork, exams, etc.
- Halt all sports & physical activities to avoid increasing your heart rate
- Avoid crowds, bright lights, & noisy public places

now, I can see that school triggered anxieties, making my symptoms even worse. School was unbearable.

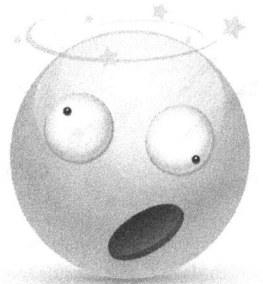

That's why every morning we had the same routine. My parents would take me to school, despite how hard I resisted, cried, hid under the bed, or tried to jump from the car on the drive there. No one knew what was wrong with me. I didn't know either. I couldn't tell them what was happening, I just knew I was different on the inside, and that I was scared. I'm not sure why I couldn't, or wouldn't, tell anyone about the lights, the noise, the slow motion, my brain's inability to focus. I felt like no one believed me.

Around me, people seemed to be everywhere, moving like crawling ants. All I could say to the doctor and my parents was "I don't know what's wrong with me." My mom begged me to describe what I was feeling and I couldn't. Honestly, I didn't know how to describe those feelings; I didn't have words for what it felt like to have my brain spinning around in my head. I couldn't remember things and people thought I was lying. Anyway, who would believe a headache and stomach ache could last this long? I could only talk to my dog, Charlie. He was the only one who *got it* and seemed to understand what was wrong and how to comfort me.

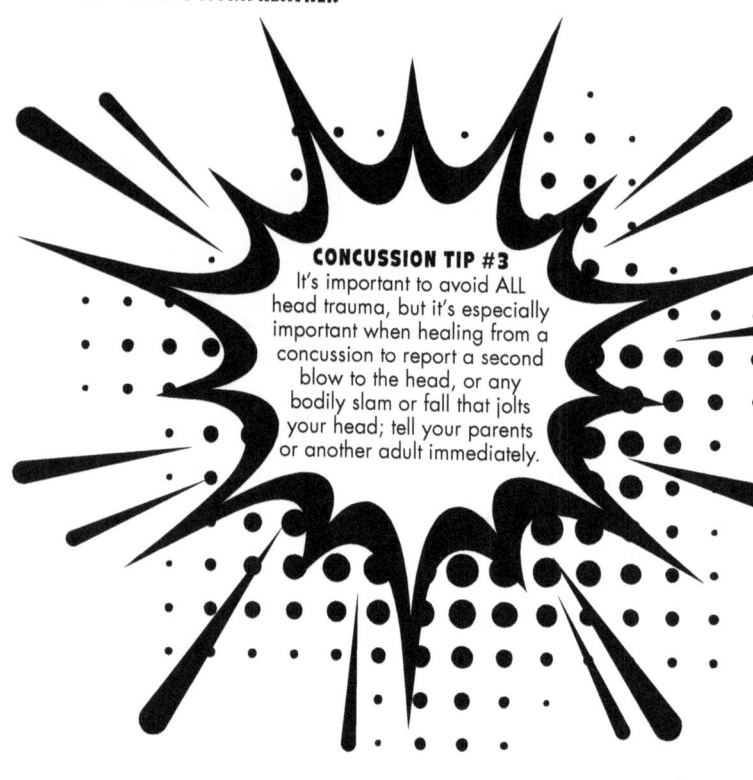

CONCUSSION TIP #3
It's important to avoid ALL head trauma, but it's especially important when healing from a concussion to report a second blow to the head, or any bodily slam or fall that jolts your head; tell your parents or another adult immediately.

Eventually my mom began talking to other people who had experienced concussions, and she began to understand that my strange behaviors were the result of a traumatic injury to my brain. Because so many people recover from concussions within a week, no one in my family had suspected brain trauma.

I still hadn't told them about the additional blows to my head from the trampoline and wrestling incidents. But the more people my mom talked to, the more she discovered that personalities can temporarily change from a concussion. We heard stories about those who

said they wanted to fight one minute and would cry the next. Issues included:
- Problems sleeping.
- Problems thinking.
- Problems with focus.
- Problems with memory.
- Headaches that wouldn't go away.
- Strange body tingling.
- Hyper-sensitivity to sounds and lights.
- Feelings of sadness.
- Irritability.
- Blurry vision.
- Dizziness and trouble with balance.
- Nausea.
- Feeling scared or nervous—uncontrollable crying.

I had all of these symptoms. I was miserable, and just riding in a car made me sick. I couldn't go to church because of the noise and the people. I ended up quitting Boy Scouts, and I couldn't play sports or hang out with my friends.

All I did was lie on the couch and worry and cry about how I couldn't go to school because of all the noise, lights, and hundreds of people. Everything at school felt brighter and louder than it should. We went to doctor after doctor, and I wasn't getting better. All I knew was that I wasn't who I used to be. And I was terrified.

One day my mom talked to a friend—a teacher who had also experienced a concussion—and discovered that it had taken her *six months* to start feeling normal again. Since my parents believed that my health was the most important thing and that rest was the best medicine, they agreed that I should stay home until I was headache-free for twenty-four hours.

The doctors provided homebound paperwork for the school, which meant that a teacher would bring work to me at home and provide lessons a few times a week.

And once I was allowed to stay home from school to rest, and away from the environment that was triggering symptoms, I slowly, *finally*, began to heal.

As I recovered, doctors would give me medication for anxiety and sleep because of the changes in my sleep pattern. One time I stayed awake for forty-eight hours straight, and it was miserable. I was screaming, "This is torture!" The medicine didn't always agree with me. One night I had hallucinations for about an hour of big, fuzzy spiders. The spiders seemed so real that I was screaming and describing how many spiders were coming at me, the size of them and the color. On another night I started making high-pitched noises and was rolling back and forth on my bed. I was out of control.

My mom helped me get to the floor, but soon I was rolling uncontrollably on the floor, and rubbing my face with my hands, slapping my face, and rubbing my face across the rugs in an attempt to remove whatever I was seeing in the hallucination. I couldn't talk, either; I could only make high-pitched noises. This particular episode lasted about thirty minutes. My parents held me and prayed.

The next day, my mom called the doctor, and he said to discontinue the medicine for a three-day period. But once I restarted the medicine, I had another repeat episode. The last episode happened on a Sunday night. Luckily the next morning we reached out to a neurologist who had been recommended by a friend from church, and we were there by nine-thirty that Monday morning.

This neurologist worked with patients who had concussions and brain injuries. He knew the best medicine for headaches. He wouldn't give me medicine for my panic attacks because of the bad side effects, so I had to go to a psychiatrist for that, and, fortunately, I didn't have any negative reactions to the headache medicine.

Sometimes I would hide my pills and not take them, because I thought they made things worse. The only medicine I wanted to take was Ibuprofen and my mom had to hide the pills because she was afraid I was going to take too many.

The neurologist wanted me to take an impact test that measures memory and reaction time. I tried to take the test, but couldn't. I couldn't even concentrate on the screens long enough to finish the simplest test.

I remember the nurse getting aggravated with me because I couldn't take the test.

The doctor explained that all of these symptoms were normal for someone who had a concussion and that over time I would get better. My CT scans and MRIs were normal. The neurologist said he'd never had a patient he couldn't help, which sounded encouraging. He also suggested that we find someone I could talk to and who could help to explain or understand what was going on inside my body. By this time, however, I was already growing angrier and angrier over the number of doctors' appointments.

This had been going on for three months and no pill or doctor seemed to help. Everyone was treating me like a baby and wouldn't let me do anything. My TV and screen time were limited. I couldn't go to school. I looked normal, I had ten toes and ten fingers, and yet

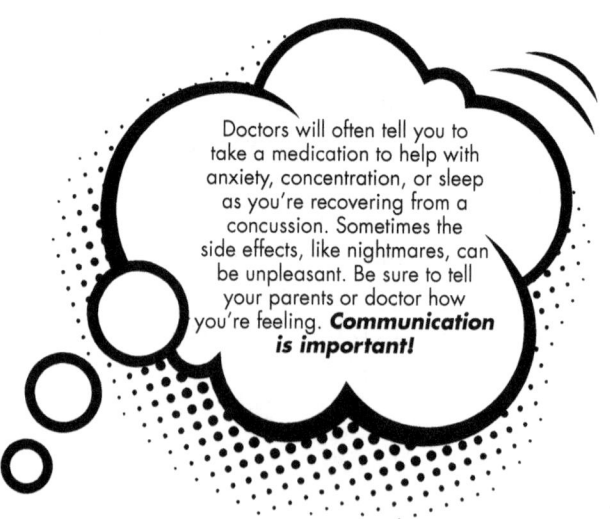

Doctors will often tell you to take a medication to help with anxiety, concentration, or sleep as you're recovering from a concussion. Sometimes the side effects, like nightmares, can be unpleasant. Be sure to tell your parents or doctor how you're feeling. **Communication is important!**

nobody, not even I, could understand or explain what was wrong or when I would feel better.

My mom was so concerned, she followed me around all the time. One minute I'd feel well enough to play with my friends, and the next, I was sick. We'd go to ball games, and I would start throwing up as soon as we got home. I remember begging to go to the annual Cleveland County Fair; I just wanted to walk around and feel normal again. But I threw up on the way home, was nauseated for days afterwards, and was so tired.

My whole life at this point consisted of lying on the couch with the covers over my head or going to doctors' appointments, which by this point included our general practitioner, a concussion specialist, a rehab therapist, an upper cervical specialist, a counselor, a massage therapist, church pastors, and a neurologist—and now this neurologist wanted to add a psychiatrist to my list.

When I resisted getting in the car one day for an appointment, my dad physically picked me up and placed me in the car. I went crazy on him, kicking and screaming and counting to 800 on the drive there. He took me home.

When we got to the psychiatrist, I just refused to talk. Here's why: *nothing was helping me,* and I couldn't understand why they wanted to give me medicine that had bad side effects. It was confusing to hear them say this medicine could help when it could also make me hurt myself, as I'd already experienced

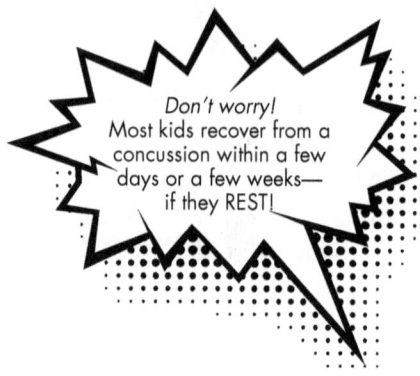

from hallucinations. This is why I would sometimes not take my pills or would hide them. Besides, all the doctors could say anyway was *no TV, no phone, no computer, and to rest, rest, rest.* I was beginning to believe I was going to feel like this for the rest of my life. I was feeling hopeless. All I could say was that there was no point, and no one could help me.

Eight months had passed and I was trying to work my way back into school. I was still mostly homebound, but I would attempt school every day for however long I could take it. I was also still terrified of the building; just seeing the red tiles of the roof from our car could set off panic. I didn't think I'd be able to do the work once I was in class. For some reason, I still couldn't explain my symptoms in a way that made sense to anyone who might have been able to help.

Then one day it occurred to me to ask my mom to make an eye appointment. I would have said something before then, but remember I was forgetful and walking around in a daze. My eye balls seemed to be bouncing around. This was another reason school was so hard. I felt like quitting, but my family kept pushing.

The eye doctor was finally the one person who understood why everything had been so hard for so long. I was seeing double and couldn't track words while reading. When I said my eyes were jumping around, she knew what that meant. I was so happy someone finally understood the problem.

From there, I began to work with her vision team twice a week. These appointments helped me to regain my confidence. I wasn't going crazy!

The fix wasn't a quick one, but over twenty-four weeks that included forty-eight appointments, I saw big improvements. The eye doctor understood the connection between the headaches and nausea. When you have problems with balance, you feel dizzy and sick to your stomach. All the reading and writing at school made me feel nauseated because of my vision problems.

Nineteen months after my concussion and the secondary blows that caused additional brain trauma, I began to feel like myself again. I had a hard time starting the seventh grade, but with the intervention of good teachers and friends, I went back for half days at first.

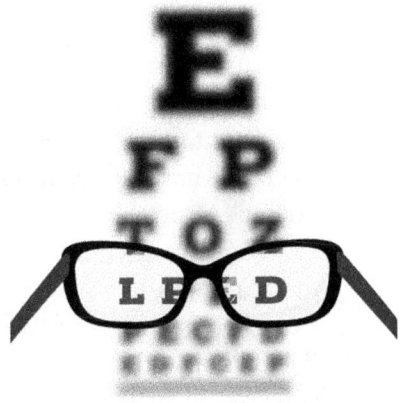

Eventually even half days turned out to be too much, so I returned for just an hour a day and slowly built up my hours from there. We finally found a counselor who had also suffered a brain injury, and this counselor helped me understand why I was so tired and slept all the time.

I am happy to say that I'm now back in school full-time. I have to take breaks sometimes, but at least I know if I take a break, it will keep me from becoming overwhelmed. The school has given me accommodations for certain things—like tests or long homework assignments—that require a little more time and concentration. I still have a real hard time taking notes, copying from the smart board, and flipping back and forth on paper.

I play golf, and I've been on the wrestling team. People judged my family for letting me wrestle and for allowing me to do other active things, but wanting to return to sports and other fun activities helps me feel normal again and feeling normal is important to your mental health recovery too. Besides, my parents wouldn't have allowed me to do anything without a doctor's approval.

Two years after my concussion and the second blow that caused additional trauma, I still love all sports! I've improved my golf game, I went 12-0 in wrestling, I've continued hunting, and discovered—thanks to the concussion—a love for fishing. My mom sometimes jokes she wants to put me inside a bubble, but the truth is, we can get hurt anywhere—riding in a car, falling at home, and doing just about anything. I'm so glad for my parents' support through all this.

I wanted to share my story to help you understand that when you're recovering from a concussion or brain trauma you can feel fine one day and feel like a different person the next.

This is normal.

And it gets better.

No one wakes up one morning deciding to be someone totally unlike who he or she was the day before. Unless you've experienced a concussion or brain injury, or cared for someone who has experienced one, you can't understand or appreciate the seriousness. Once people began to believe I was telling the truth about not feeling well and not making up things to get out of going to school, I began to improve.

Part of the problem, too, was my inability to describe what I was actually feeling. Maybe this inability was related to the injury, itself. I tend to believe so since I'd never had communication problems before the concussion, and haven't since reaching this phase of my recovery. Looking back I believe it is normal to be scared when your brain feels like it's spinning around inside your head.

This is why I think it's important for you to know about my story, and how I finally recovered. If you ever suspect you have a concussion, or get diagnosed with one, be as honest as possible with yourself and your family.

AT HOME

STAGE 1:	**STAGE 2:**	
PHYSICAL & COGNITIVE REST • Basic board games, crafts, talk on phone • Activities that do not increase heart rate or break a sweat **Limit/Avoid:** • Computer, TV, texting, video games, reading **No:** • School work • Sports • Work • Driving until cleared by a health care professional	**START WITH LIGHT COGNITIVE ACTIVITY:** Gradually increase cognitive activity up to 30 min. Take frequent breaks. **Prior activities plus:** • Reading, TV, drawing • Limited peer contact and social networking Contact school to create *Return to School* plan. **No:** • School attendance • Sports • Work	**WHEN LIGHT COGNITIVE ACTIVITY IS TOLERATED:** Introduce school work. **Prior activities plus:** • School work as per *Return to School* plan Communicate with school on student's progression.
REST	**GRADUALLY ADD COGNITIVE ACTIVITY INCLUDING SCHOOL WORK AT HOME**	
When symptoms start to improve OR after resting for 2 days max, BEGIN STAGE 2.	Tolerates 30 min. of cognitive activity, introduce school work at home.	Tolerates 60 min. of school work in two 30 min. intervals, BEGIN STAGE 3.

STAGE 6: FULL-TIME SCHOOL:
Full days at school, no learning accommodations.
• Attend all classes
• All homework
• Full extracurricular involvement
• All testing

Adapted from the Return to Learn protocol by G.F. Strong School Program (Vancouver School Board) Adolescent and Young Adult Program, G.F. Strong Rehabilitation Centre.

If you don't, and continue too soon with physical activities and school work, you're risking permanent brain damage, even death. You'll probably get tired of hearing that rest is the only cure. I sure did. But it's true: *Rest is the only cure.* And you probably

AT SCHOOL

STAGE 3:
BACK TO SCHOOL PART-TIME:
Part-time school with maximum accommodations.
Prior activities plus:
- School work at school as per *Return to School* Plan

No:
- P.E., physical activity at lunch/recess, homework, testing, sports, assemblies, field trips

Communicate with school on student's progression.

SCHOOL WORK ONLY AT SCHOOL

Tolerates 120 min. of cognitive activity in 30-45 min. intervals, BEGIN STAGE 4

STAGE 4:
PART-TIME SCHOOL:
Increase school time with moderate accommodations.
Prior activities plus:
- Increase time at school
- Decrease accomodations
- Homework-up to 30 min./day
- Classroom testing with adaptations

No:
- P.E., physical activity at lunch/recess, sports, standardized testing

Communicate with school on student's progression.

INCREASE SCHOOL WORK, INTRODUCE HOMEWORK, DECREASE LEARNING ACCOMMODATIONS

Tolerates 240 min. of cognitive activity in 45-60 min. intervals, BEGIN STAGE 5

STAGE 5:
FULL-TIME SCHOOL:
Full days at school, minimal accommodations.
Prior activities plus:
- Start to eliminate accommodations
- Increase homework to 60 min./day
- Limit routine testing to one test per day with adaptations

No:
- P.E., physical activity at lunch/recess, sports, standardized testing

WORK UP TO FULL DAYS AT SCHOOL, MINIMAL LEARNING ACCOMMODATIONS

Tolerates school full-time with no learning accommodations BEGIN STAGE 6

STAGE 6 (CONT.):
No:
- Full participation in P.E. or sports until *Return to Sports* protocol completed and written medical clearance provided

FULL ACADEMIC LOAD

Return to School protocol completed focus on *RETURN TO SPORTS*

won't like it any more than I did, because rest without TV or video games is boring. But slowing down your brain activity, along with identifying and avoiding your triggers, are the only ways your brain can heal itself after a concussion. The more you rest immediately after a concussion, the sooner you'll be back to normal and doing all the things you want to do.

Besides, what's a few weeks of rest compared to a year or two?

PART II
MYRA HEAVNER

A MOTHER'S STORY

Because we live near Charlotte, North Carolina, we attend Carolina Panthers football games. So when Luke wanted to play football, his father and I agreed and signed him up.

Like many parents, we hoped our son would enjoy all the benefits that come with learning how to be a dependable teammate. Most of all, we hoped for an injury-free experience.

Even now, two and a half years after Luke's first concussion, I want to make it clear that I'm not sharing our family's journey through concussion recovery as a way to shame parents who encourage their children to play football or any other youth collision sports activity such as soccer, lacrosse, hockey, boxing, wrestling, and baseball. Even the sports we don't typically associate with concussions—the lesser collision sports such as tennis, golf, basketball, swimming, and volleyball—can still produce a concussion from a head blow after a hard fall or a blow to the head from a ball, racket, club, or elbow.

While a hefty part of this book noticeably includes information related to youth sports injuries, the reality is that Luke and I could just as well be writing it due to a concussion he suffered from a stumble at home—or as you may have learned by reading his story, from a variety of different mishaps. I wouldn't have been any more prepared to identify a concussion had one occurred in our home than Luke's actual concussions that happened during football practice and on a trampoline less than two weeks before the start of sixth grade.

My intent here is twofold: to provide what I hope will be valuable information should you ever suspect your child might have suffered a concussion; and to help you help your child prevent concussions in the first place. And because the number of concussions each year resulting from youth sports activities is second to motor vehicle accidents, Luke and I thought the additional information we've included here related to concussion prevention in youth sports could be helpful. We've also separated our stories into Parts I and II so that you, the parent, can choose how much information you think your child is ready to absorb about concussions.

Look, concussions are hateful, and when a concussion and a subsequent injury invaded my son's mind and body, the brain trauma put him in a dark storm for nearly two years. A concussion is not only a hardship on the patient, but a hardship on the entire family. I hope our family's story will unify other families and provide support for weathering the storm that potentially lies ahead.

Without the support of my family, friends, and co-workers, I could have easily lost my job, business, and marriage during Luke's recovery from concussions. Most of the time, I battled with feelings of guilt, grief, confusion, and helplessness. What parent wants to face that she's unable to provide her child with answers?

Please remember this: when it comes to concussions, not even the experts have all the answers.

So, here's *my* story:

When Luke first told us about the hard hit he'd taken at football practice, he complained of a headache and went to bed. We expected him to be fine by morning. But he wasn't, and so we sought medical attention. This was when we discovered that he'd suffered a concussion. Our doctor said Luke was expected to improve within a few days. Treatment included rest

---

UNDERSTANDING THE TWO PHYSICAL FORCES THAT LEAD TO CONCUSSIONS & BRAIN INURIES

- The first type of force that leads to concussion and brain injury is linear force. Imagine two young athletes in a head-on helmet impact—this is linear force. But since most concussions actually happen in motor vehicle accidents, a better example might be a head-on collision with another object—another car, a guardrail, a concrete wall, a tree. The collision forces a violent front-to-back jolt, causing the brain to smack hard against the rough, bony interior of the head. For children under fourteen, these injuries are particularly dangerous because their brains are not protected by myelin coating until their teenaged years.

- Second is rotational force. This is what we believe first happened to Luke—a face-masking injury that was then coupled with the hard blow of his head to the ground. Because Luke couldn't anticipate the face mask and the brunt of the blow; his head was whipped from one direction to the opposite one. When the brain smacks against the skull by a rotational force, the brain can stretch, tearing blood vessels and tissue, as well as what is torn from the blow against the rough, bony skull.

and Tylenol or Motrin for his headache. He was to rest until he was headache-free for twenty-four hours. Luke was suffering from what I now know as classic concussion symptoms—headache, everything moving in slow motion, fogginess, and excessive sleepiness.

When the headaches worsened, doctors said there was nothing more they could do unless Luke began to throw up, and he didn't during this early phase. But the headaches continued to worsen.

Most often MRI or CT scans only show brain bleeds; they don't show the effects of a concussion. Luke's scans appeared normal.

After eight days of acting dazed and lying around, Luke told us he was headache-free. We believed him. I wish I had been more skeptical, but we had been so worried for days that I think we got caught up in relief that he could resume his normal activities.

I didn't realize until it was too late that after you get one concussion, you're more likely and more susceptible to get a second concussion, and that the second blow can cause permanent brain damage or even be deadly. Luke was just eleven at the time when he suffered the face masking, whiplash jolt, and hard tackle at football practice. He didn't report the hit to his coaches because his coaches hadn't warned their young players

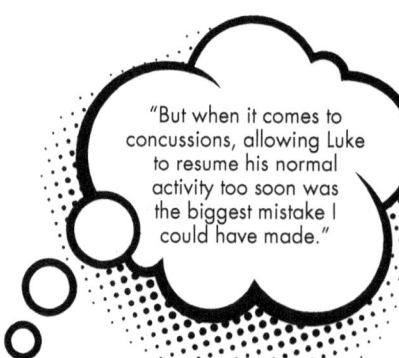

"But when it comes to concussions, allowing Luke to resume his normal activity too soon was the biggest mistake I could have made."

> **IF YOUR CHILD PLAYS YOUTH SPORTS:**
>
> Has your child's coach received concussion training? Many youth athletic teams are coached by well-meaning volunteers, often parents of the players on their team, who have little to no knowledge about concussion symptoms. If this is the case for your child's team, please speak up. Encourage all coaches to receive concussion training, or be extra vigilant about observing your child's behavior during and after practices and games.

about concussions and concussion symptoms. When Luke was hit, he was expected to jump back into play, as were all the kids, with the no-pain-no-gain attitude you might expect from professional athletes. Not even professional athletes, however, are immune to concussions. Most times, at this age, coaches are parent volunteers with no training on the dangers and symptoms of concussions.

Luke was like most eleven-year-old boys: full of energy, with little fear when it came to running, jumping, wrestling, swimming, riding bikes, or anything else that involved a ball. So the first thing Luke wanted to do when he was supposedly headache-free was tag along with a friend to a football practice weigh-in.

After the weigh-in, the boys went to a friend's birthday party since school was going to start in a few days.

When I picked Luke up from the party that night, he jumped in the car and was crying and screaming that his head was on fire. I asked all sorts of questions, but no one at the party, including Luke, told me that he'd hit his head while on the trampoline or had been accidentally kicked in the head while wrestling with a friend. At home he went to bed. The next morning, we began a nineteen-month journey of hell.

The headaches, he told us, had returned. The headaches began mostly in the front of his forehead and wrapped around his ears to the back of his head. His personality changed drastically, too, and all he could answer to every question was, "I don't know." His pupils were enormous and he appeared dazed, as if enshrouded in a mental fog. His father and I were baffled.

On the tenth day since the original face-masking injury, our family prepared for the first day of school. Luke was dressed but looked nervous. His nervousness seemed natural at the time because he was about to start middle school. By the time we reached the school, his nervousness had drastically increased. At the time, I had no idea that anxiety or nervousness was a classic symptom of a concussion.

But when Luke voiced how badly he hurt, I rushed him to the emergency room, and this was when doctors confirmed that Luke still had a concussion. Luke was supposed to rest, they told me, until he was *headache-free for twenty-four hours*. No one informed us that recovery could take weeks, months, or even years for the symptoms to disappear. We were referred to a concussion specialist too.

What I wouldn't discover for another several months is that Luke had received additional blows from the fall on the trampoline and the accidental kick to his head, and that those head traumas were leading to serious brain injury. According to youth concussion expert and adviser to the NFL, Dr. Robert Cantu, in his book, *Concussions and Our Kids: America's Leading Expert On How To Protect Young Athletes and Keep Sports Safe,* written with Mark Hyman, "Concussions ... trigger a complicated chain of chemical and metabolic reactions, which are known as the neurometabolic cascade of concussion."

This process, according to Cantu, creates confusion. No longer is the brain properly relaying signals and messages.

Adds Cantu, "From being pushed and pulled violently, the brain goes into an overactive state, a state of hyperalertness, releasing chemicals called neurotransmitters. These are the chemicals needed for one cell to communicate with the next. In this situation, the cells begin communicating in a disorderly way, blasting out impulses to all cells at the

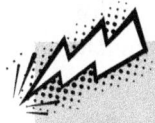

DR. CANTU'S FOUR MAJOR CATEGORIES OF CONCUSSION SYMPTOMS:

1. **SOMATIC:** Headaches, nausea, vomiting, balance and/or visual problems, dizzy spells, and issues such as sensitivity to light and noise.
2. **EMOTIONAL:** Sadness to the point of depression (even suicide), nervousness, and irritability.
3. **SLEEP DISTURBANCE:** Sleeping more or less than usual and trouble falling asleep.
4. **COGNITIVE:** Difficulty concentrating, troubles with memory, feeling mentally slow or as if in a fog that will not lift.

> **TIPS FOR IDENTIFYING A CONCUSSION:**
>
> - After sports practices and games, ask your child specifics—who won the game, the score, the color of the jerseys worn by the opposing team—instead of "How do you feel?"
> - Recite a handful of numbers or letters, or several whole words, and ask your child to repeat them, and try again, reversing the order. Make a game of it. A few minutes later, ask your child to repeat the numbers, letters, or words. Memory loss and confusion can be symptoms of a concussion.
> - Listen for concussion clues in words or phrases such as dazed ... my head hurts ... everything is too loud ... sick to my stomach ... my fingers (or feet) are numb (or tingling).
> - Watch your child for issues related to physical balance.

same time so that the system becomes overloaded. At this point, the brain loses its ability to regulate certain chemical balances."

Three days later, I drove Luke to the concussion specialist recommended by the doctors at the emergency room. The concussion specialist also advised Luke to take the rest of the week off from school, to rest, and to return to school on Monday with a medical follow-up after school. We followed the doctor's orders even though they conflicted with the six-stage *Return to Learn* advice we'd received from the emergency room medical team.

And this is where I believe everything began to unravel and eventually prolong Luke's concussion symptoms. The concussion specialist hadn't even mentioned the six-stage program, and I didn't think to question his medical orders at this point. I thought everything was going to be fine in a couple of days. No one had mentioned how serious this could be. So on Monday—*day 18 since the original injury*—I drove Luke back to school, despite his constant protests and crying.

My mistake, *again*. I should not have allowed Luke to return to school. I should have followed the advice of the emergency room doctors, or at least questioned the confliction of their medical advice with that of the concussion specialist.

My husband and I made Luke return to school because he had a follow-up appointment with the concussion specialist, that day anyway.

During the second appointment, the concussion specialist conducted a few simple tests with Luke. In one of these, the doctor revealed flash cards with simple three- or four-letter words. After a few seconds, the doctor removed the card and asked Luke to recite the word. Flashcard after flashcard appeared and disappeared, and Luke couldn't recall a single word or letter. He had no memory.

For a second test, Luke was to follow the movement of the doctor's finger. When Luke couldn't even follow the doctor's simple finger test, the doctor glanced over at me with a stunned expression. The doctor asked me if Luke had always struggled with school, hinting that perhaps Luke's problems were related to his being a delayed learner or intellectually challenged in some way. I told him no, that Luke in fact had been a good student until this injury. I can still feel the frustration of that moment. I shrugged my shoulders, threw up my hands, thinking, *You're the doctor, for crying out loud ... I don't know what's going on!*

When I mentioned the concussion to a good friend of mine who was also a teacher, she suggested I immediately request a 504 plan for Luke from the concussion specialist, and that I needed his recommendation. The doctor's response was that we were too early in Luke's recovery process to request a 504 plan.

504 plans are formal plans that schools develop to give kids with disabilities the support they need. These plans prevent discrimination and protect the rights of kids with disabilities in school. They're covered under Section 504 of the Rehabilitation Act, which is a civil rights law.

We were sent away with doctor's orders that released Luke from school for the rest of the week, but that also said Luke was to return to school the following week. There was no mention of the importance of being headache-free for twenty-four hours first, as we'd heard from the ER doctors.

So that week I met with Luke's teachers to get his work, and they told me not to worry about the school work. They'd had other students who had suffered concussions, and so they understood that a protocol of rest, no lights, and no school was best for Luke.

Despite weeks of Luke's inability to sustain whole days in school, the principal and school counselor insisted that if Luke would just get a full week under his belt, he'd be fine. To be fair, this was Luke's first year at middle school with new teachers, a new principal, and a new counselor. Luke didn't know these people, so it might make sense to think his problems were related to anxiety over the new environment. But they weren't.

Throughout this journey I'd discover a slew of popular, actually harmful, myths that swirled around the topic of concussions—the most popular myth being how others who'd had their "bells rung" had been cured after a good night's sleep, so shouldn't everyone? And there were the particularly insensitive comments such as: *I couldn't sleep at night if my kid couldn't go to school ... this is a mental illness right?* And, *Must be really bad if the doctors just write your kid out of school, he looks fine to me.* And, *Luke's behavior is normal for a teenager, they can't keep up with anything.* Surprisingly some even claimed that Luke didn't have a brain injury, and that he'd probably never graduate high school. One nurse even said, "I couldn't deal with having a concussed kid." By this point, we were feeling unfairly judged, and as if we had somehow become the moving targets for anyone's release of insensitivity. What most fail to

---

DR. ROBERT CANTU, LEADING YOUTH CONCUSSION EXPERT AND ADVISER TO THE NFL:

"There is no 'normal' recovery for a child with a concussion—no timeline or timetable to predict when symptoms will lift. Symptoms can last for weeks or months, or in a few cases, years. Some kids will have to leave school for a year. Others have to give up one collision sport they enjoy, or even worse, all competitive sports."

> **THE BEST THERAPY FOR RECOVERING FROM A CONCUSSION IS**
> # REST!
>
> We couldn't expect Luke to do nothing all day. That was unreasonable. But we learned by trial and error to limit the activities that overstressed his cognitive abilities, causing him to relapse into headaches and other severe concussion symptoms.
>
> TV watching, computer screen time, test-taking, texting, and social media usage had to be restricted and slowly increased or decreased, depending upon his progress.

understand is that there is no one-size-fits-all when it comes to concussions that can develop from a number of variables: the type of blow to the head; the age of the patient; and the patient's immediate response after the blow to the head.

The *next biggest mistake* I made was in not listening to my gut instincts; no one knows your child better than you. I should have insisted on a conference with the doctor and the school because I knew that, despite what the principal or counselor believed, Luke's anxiety was not related to middle-school angst. Luke's behavior was not normal; this was not my son.

My son had been at the top of his game for fifth grade. He had improved his math and reading skills over the summer by working with a pastor who was a math genius and tutor. Luke had been excited about the start of sixth grade. He'd designed and ordered his own Nike ID shoes, which had to be the shade of red that matched his new school's colors, and had to include his name. A friend had embroidered the school mascot—a chief—on Luke's book bag.

When Luke kept crying and protesting about going to school, I was most worried that he'd fall behind. The more he protested, the more I pushed for what I believed was his benefit. I didn't know, of course, at the time that Luke's growing anxiety issues were related to his concussion, and that he still hadn't told us about the second injury—the one we later discovered could have killed him.

I did keep a journal about Luke's behavior—mostly his anxiety issues related to mood, appetite, and sleep, as well as other symptoms that could possibly lead to the discovery of a pattern. At the time we were in the thick of it all, every day seemed to give birth to a new symptom from a new trigger. So many triggers, so many symptoms—the journaling helped to keep track of them all. Days without eating, sleepless nights, and days of too much sleep. The journal also became a useful roadmap that I would give to doctors to read so Luke wouldn't have to recall and relive his misery. As it was, Luke was changing every day before our eyes, and we were frightened. It's only natural for a parent to wonder when, and if, her child will recover.

Eventually I learned by talking to others who had suffered concussions, not from the concussion specialist or Luke's doctors, that anxiety is an actual symptom, and that some of the more obvious triggers for anxiety are noise, lights, and crowds. Another trigger was Luke's inability to concentrate on his school work. My doctor explained to me how severe concussions can be. He also discussed possible emotional side effects and put me in touch with other parents who were dealing with simliar situations. This was very helpful to me.

In some ways I'm sure I was in shock, or denial, that my previously normal, well-adjusted son was becoming a stranger to me. He would cry, get angry, and then break out into sudden laughter. He had bad reactions to several medications that included seizure-like behavior, forgetfulness. He couldn't remember where he'd put anything, and would sometimes put his shoes on the wrong feet. He moved throughout his days in a fog. One day he'd appear fine, and we'd think he was back to normal; the next day he couldn't get off the couch. He couldn't concentrate. You could tell the wires to his brain were uncontrollably live-zapping his emotions. People kept saying he looked fine, I called that the brave face, but outsiders didn't see what we saw. I could tell others thought he wasn't being truthful because he would joke and appear fine, while texting me he was miserable. He did look normal, but he wasn't the old Luke, he became the new Luke.

And then the depression set in. He would curl up in a ball in the shower for long periods of time and sleep most of the day. I remember trying to make him keep a schedule and would bring him to work with me and he would crawl up under a desk and sleep for hours. I would ask teachers, coaches, or anyone

> **CONCUSSION GLOSSARY**
>
>
>
> - **CONCUSSION**: a violent shaking of the brain from a blow to the head or from a sudden rotational change of direction. Concussions generally happen as the result of linear or rotational forces that cause the brain to hit the rough inside of the skull. It is a dangerous myth to assume that one hasn't suffered concussion unless one has been knocked unconscious.
> - **POST-CONCUSSION SYDROME**: a term used to describe concussions that last much longer than the usual two- to three-week recovery time, and that are accompanied with unusually intense symptoms.
> - **SECOND IMPACT SYNDROME**: a condition, sometimes fatal, in which the brain swells from a second blow to the head before the first concussion has fully healed.
> - **CHRONIC TRAUMATIC ENCEPHALOPATHY**: CTE is a degenerative brain disease that can occur after repetitive brain trauma. CTE has been discovered in children as young as seventeen. Researchers believe children under twelve who suffer head trauma, such as concussions, are more susceptive to CTE than children who suffer head trauma over the age of twelve.

to let him assist or help be part of the team, just to try and get him off the couch and make him feel a part or be involved with all the things he used to love. Luke would say, "No, what's the point? I will never get better," or, "I will be like this the rest of my life." Each day our goal was to have Luke take one more step than the day before and prayed he could endure another minute longer without any symptoms.

While all this madness was happening, I was still trying to get his work from the school to keep him current. One afternoon I asked a former teacher of Luke's to work with him, and she said, "Myra, shut him down. He is wound up." She understood about concussion symptoms and recovery because she'd walked this path during her daughter's concussion recovery process.

I also sought advice from another friend who had actually suffered a concussion, and who was a teacher. "When I fell and hit my head," she said, "I wanted to fight my kids and my husband. I even tried to take my clothes off in the doctor's office. I couldn't control my emotions. Take Luke out of school until he is able."

That's when Luke's father and I realized that Luke's mental health, not academics, was our priority. For Luke's sake, we placed him on *homebound,* a program that allowed Luke to work from home and to receive his lessons from one teacher, and because of Luke's anxieties, the principal and counselor suggested we take Luke to school for a few hours a day when he felt up to it. We knew as soon as Luke was able he would catch up. And frankly, we were all more than a little exhausted from Luke's crying protests every day when it was time to go to school.

Church for Luke had also become a problem. He couldn't handle the crowd, the music, any of the noise. We spoke with the daughter of a family at our church who had suffered several concussions. She told us to listen to Luke. "If he can't go, he can't go," she said. "Trust what he says." This was when I truly noticed the triggers to his anxiety—the large groups of people and loud noises.

Another painful mistake we made as parents during this journey was that we'd begun to label him as lazy.

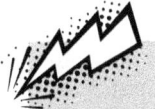

> **DID YOU KNOW?**
>
> The Center for Injury Research in Columbus, Ohio, reports that more high school soccer players suffered concussions in 2010 than basketball, baseball, wrestling, and softball players combined. That same year, female soccer players suffered 25,953 concussions, and male players 20,247 concussions. Compare that to basketball—boys logged 11,013 concussions.
>
> (Reported in *Concussions and Our Kids* by Dr. Robert Cantu and Mark Hyman.)

My husband and the rest of our family couldn't wrap our heads around why Luke couldn't attend school, yet he could tolerate other things, such as fishing or being with friends. Luke always said, "Don't you know I would rather be at school than stay at home?" His Grandma, who was a retired teacher, would stay with him day after day and would read to him while he lay with the covers over his head.

We begged him and bribed Luke, and when those tactics didn't work, we punished him. We tried various medications, and finally gave up on those after witnessing our son's frightening episodes of hallucinations. Luke would always tell me, "I don't believe in pills, Momma," and during housecleaning, I'd find his medicine strewn all over the house. What I eventually had to accept was that there was no solution for Luke's sudden personality change be it begging, bribes, punishment, or pills. We would have to learn to cope with and love the stranger who was now living in our home. I could see in his eyes that he didn't understand why this was happening to him.

In my opinion, the only cures for a concussion and post-concussion syndrome are to rest and carefully follow the six stages of *Return to Learn*, as well as to avoid stressful triggers or activities that aggravate symptoms. The period of rest must be extended until

HOW TO PREVENT MORE CONCUSSIONS IN YOUTH COLLISION SPORTS

- Encourage children to play flag football until they're fourteen, when their neck muscles are more developed to support their heads and their brains more mature and protected by myelin coating. Every hard tackle or violent jolt to the body after concussion can develop into the degenerative brain disease, CTE, by adulthood, although CTE has already been discovered in the brains of college-aged victims. The parents of NFL quarterback Tom Brady wouldn't allow their son to play tackle football until he was fourteen!
- Encourage youth football coaches to adopt a hit count policy during practices and games the way baseball youth coaches employ the pitch count.
- Encourage the use of helmets for lacrosse players. While helmets offer limited protection, some protection is better than none.
- Discourage heading in soccer until fourteen for the same reasons. According to soccer and medical experts, soccer practices that involve multiple kicks from coaches or parents directly at players for heading are unnecessary—even irresponsible.
- Discourage youth baseball players from sliding headfirst into bases. Helmets offer limited protection and often fall off during a run. Adding chin straps to youth helmets would be another plus toward concussion prevention, and some youth leagues are now requiring chin straps.
- Discourage body checking in hockey until after the age of fourteen for all the same reasons as described above.
- Discourage any attitude that rewards children for inflicting, or playing through, pain.
- Do not tolerate head butts in any sport.
- According to *Sports Health May/June 2013* less than 1% of young athletes aged 6-17 move on to achieve elite status in basketball, soccer, baseball, softball, or football. It is not worth risking your child's future health and wellness for any game.

your child is headache- and symptom-free. For most concussion patients, relief comes within a few days. For others, a few weeks. We were months in, however, before we finally understood the severity of Luke's situation and we never dreamed it would be such a long recovery process. Still, every day I remained optimistic, thinking he would be better.

To ensure Luke was following all instructions, physical activities and hang-outs with friends were monitored. I was relentless. I did my best to ensure he was actually lying on the couch, resting, because if you didn't keep your eye on him he would be at the neighbor's house, jumping on the trampoline, riding a hover board or bike, playing basketball—all just wanting to be a normal kid. The only time he seemed happy was when he was with friends, fishing, or eating snow cones. As a parent, you want to do everything right, but you can only restrict and demand so much before total rebellion sets in, or something much worse. Keep in mind, too, that he was a preteen going through puberty.

So, when Luke desperately wanted to go to the annual county fair, we gave in. When he wanted to take a snow cone challenge and eat a hundred snow cones, one of each flavor during a single season, we went along with it. He needed to feel normal and we were willing to do whatever it took to help him feel that way.

But on the day of the fair it was hot, and we had to park a long way from the entrance. After a while,

Luke asked us to buy him honey. I didn't know at the time he wanted the honey because he was feeling nauseated. On the drive home, we pulled over several times because of Luke's violent vomiting. For several days after the fair, he was out cold with exhaustion.

Another time, he wanted so badly to attend a Carolina Panthers football game. We relented. On the way home, however, he said he didn't feel good and became sick again. This became the routine whenever he did anything before he was fully recovered through rest.

If he went to a friend's house, he would return home feeling fine for a while. Soon after, the vomiting would begin and the concussion symptoms would worsen. We finally found a counselor who had suffered a brain injury, and who explained the effects of exhaustion, as well as how physical and mental stress contributes to exhaustion and how panic attacks affect the body. The counselor encouraged us to listen to Luke and ensure he got plenty of rest.

As a parent, I thought Luke was improving every time he was playing and having fun, but that was not the case. Physical and mental activity would often trigger symptoms, thereby prolonging any chance of a full recovery. Then his father and I would get upset when Luke played but couldn't do the things

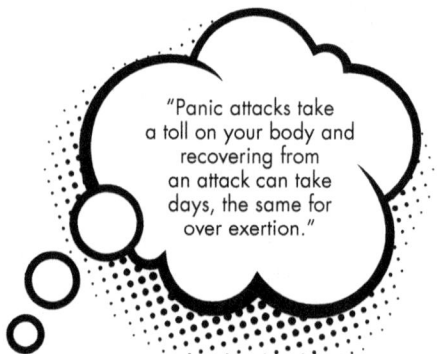

"Panic attacks take a toll on your body and recovering from an attack can take days, the same for over exertion."

we thought he should be able to do, like volunteer at church and go to school. The more we pushed, the more our assertive attitudes would trigger panic attacks that sent him to bed for days. The counselor stressed to us that the panic attacks contributed to other symptoms, and that it was important for us, and Luke, to remember that you are who you are today, not who you were yesterday, or who you will be tomorrow.

Today my advice to parents is to seek out others who have experienced and recovered from concussions; allow their experiences to fill the communication gaps between you and your child, especially if your child is unable or too frightened to adequately describe the scary symptoms or triggers that set them off.

One day, nine months after the face-masking and whiplash incident at football practice, Luke came to me and said, "I can't see. It's my vision." Finally, after all these months Luke could point us in a direction to give him the help he needed. Our eye doctor had treated Luke when he was younger for eye/hand coordination issues along with other issues related to his fine motor skills. She had tests that she could use to compare to his current abilities, and this was when all the puzzle pieces of this concussion mystery suddenly fell into place.

Luke's eye doctor was able to relate to Luke and his symptoms because of her extensive experience with other concussion patients. After an examination and the comparison of Luke's previous tests to his current abilities, she concluded that Luke was suffering from double vision and accommodative insufficiency. His ocular system, she said, had become disabled.

One recommendation from the medical community is to require all children who play collision sports undergo a battery of baseline testing on memory, vision, and balance so that these results can be compared to test results after a suspected concussion, CT scans and MRIs rarely reveal the tiny tears that can suddenly wreak havoc on a child's cognitive abilities, while these baseline tests can. However, one argument, and there are several, against the baseline testing requirement is that testing a child with a concussion can actually worsen the child's condition and slow recovery. Baseline testing should be conducted prior to the start of sports each school year.

Discovering that Luke had serious vision problems sounded scary, but hopeful. The eye doctor, however, had solutions that began with a comprehensive plan: for twenty-four weeks, Luke would receive vision therapy twice a week.

I've learned throughout this journey that support, love, and understanding were as essential to Luke's recovery as the doctor's mandatory order of *rest*. At times our family was too caught up in what others were thinking about us—the family with the son who suddenly refused to get off the couch for school.

Their misperceptions floated throughout our various social communities and felt hurtful. But I also understand how all this must have looked to outsiders. In the beginning, we felt like outsiders too.

Today Luke is completely medication free. He is back in school and can play with his friends. Eight months after his concussion injuries, Luke wanted to learn how to play golf and he joined the local junior golf program. He was looking for a new sport or hobby, and golf seemed safe. At first, Luke wanted to rent a cart. I told him he needed to walk like all the other kids do. In hindsight, I should have driven him on the golf cart and not worried about the outside perception. Trust is so important. His father and I were trying not to judge, but we were just as challenged, ourselves, with the perception of Luke being different, or of him having different needs.

This year, Luke tells me that playing golf is much easier now, and that he has no trouble walking the course and carrying his clubs. Luke's life at school has become much easier too. With the help of a few accommodations, he's now able to take tests that he wouldn't have been able to take last year.

Now when I hear that someone has a concussion, I urge them to talk with others who have recovered from one. Doctors are necessary, of course, but finding the right fit isn't always as easy as you might think. We met with many doctors who possessed all the right credentials but who weren't compassionate enough about our dilemma to help us find the root cause of Luke's continuing symptoms or explain them in a manner that hit home to us. Some doctors even scolded Luke; they called him rude and uncooperative when they couldn't fit their concussion template around his narrative. I also highly recommend that if one doctor or counselor doesn't seem to fit, be persistent about finding a doctor you feel comfortable with; don't give up.

When Luke was first injured I mentioned to our pastor how stressful it was for Luke and his Dad and I to go to all these doctors appointments because we really wouldn't get any answers except come back in six weeks and let's see how he's doing. I also worried when Luke would refuse to go into the doctor's office once we arrived for an appointment. Other times he would go in and shut down and not speak when the doctor arrived. Our pastor asked me if all those doctors were necessary. Looking back, they probably were not necessary, but we were doing what we thought was in Luke's best interest.

One of Luke's counselors complained to me about his behavior. I asked if she'd ever dealt with brain injuries and she said no. Later that week, she called with an apology. She'd researched brain injuries, and Luke's symptoms matched his behavior. She added that her son had been hit by a car at a young age and that she'd struggled with his behavior ever since. Looking back, she realized that he'd likely suffered a concussion and she'd judged and punished him unfairly.

We didn't learn about the additional blows to Luke's head after his concussion—the blows that could have killed him—until three months after the mishaps at his friend's home. This was when we were finally able to put together more pieces to his challenging recovery.

I believe Luke's first concussion might have taken a couple of weeks to recover, but the undiagnosed second blow or blows made his brain injury so much worse, though they thankfully did not kill him. Add to this our lack of knowledge about concussions, triggers, symptoms, and post-concussion syndrome … and you can see why Luke and I feel compelled to share our story. If we help only one family through this, all that we endured will have been worth it. At the time Luke had his concussion there were no celebrities or professional athletes speaking out on the issue. When NASCAR drivers and other professional athletes began to speak up and share their experiences on social media, people began to listen.

As Luke recovered, I still found it difficult not to overstress about his activities. We continued to trust Luke and to follow his lead. When half-days at school were too much, we tried home schooling, but this wasn't the best fit for Luke. Luke loves his friends and his school and always reminded us he would have rather been at school with his friends. Restrictions on computer and television time were slowly lifted as Luke's condition allowed. Physical activities like golf, wrestling, being with friends, and even participating as the ball boy for the football team, eventually returned to Luke's life, and we faced harsh judgments about these.

No one can live happily under a constant shadow of fear. Our children can get hurt in a number of ways just walking around at home, much less all the ways they can get hurt when they leave home. I find strength in my faith, family, and in prayer. Whatever arises, I love and trust that I can't always understand the mystery behind it all.

WORKS CITED

Andruszkow H, Deniz E, Urner J, et al. *Physical and psychological long-term outcome after brain injury in children and adult patients.* Health and Quality of Life Outcomes, 12 (2014).

Asemota AO, George BP, Bowman SM, et al. *Causes and trends in traumatic brain injury for United States adolescents.* J Neurotrauma, 15: 67-75 (2013).

Cantu, Robert M.D. and Hyman, Mark. *Concussions and Our Kids: America's Leading Expert On How To Protect Young Athletes And Keep Sports Safe.* Houghton Mifflin Harcourt. NY, 2012.

Centers for Disease Control and Prevention. *"Injury Prevention and Control: Traumatic Brain Injury and Concussion."* https://www.cdc.gov/traumaticbraininjury/get_the_facts.html

G.F. Strong Rehabilitation Centre. *Return to Learn protocol.* G.F. Strong School Program (Vancouver School Board) Adolescent and Young Adult Program.

Science Direct. http://www.sciencedirect.com/topics/neuroscience/second-impact-syndrome.

www.ingramcontent.com/pod-product-compliance
Lightning Source LLC
Chambersburg PA
CBHW071416040426
42444CB00009B/2274